15 Simple Ways To Lower Your Blood Pressure Naturally After 40 Without Complicated Diets

Dr. Chio Ugochukwu

15 Simple Ways To Lower Your Blood Pressure Naturally After 40 Without Complicated Diets

Published by Compass International

44546 Orchard Lane, Lancaster CA 93534

ISBN-13: 978-1514390276

ISBN-10: 1514390272

Printed in the United States of America

15 Simple Ways To Lower Your Blood Pressure Naturally After 40 Without Complicated Diets

Disclaimer

This book contains information that is based on the research, professional experience, opinions and ideas of its author. It is solely for informational and educational purposes and should not be regarded as a substitute for professional medical treatment. This is a book for people who want practical suggestions that will help them live healthier and happier lives. No information contained in this book should be considered as physical, psychological, medical, financial, tax or legal advice. The author and publisher assume no liability or responsibility for any adverse consequences for the use of any product, information, idea or instruction contained in the content provided to you through this book. Always consult your healthcare provider first.

Dedication

This book is dedicated to those who struggle to control their high blood pressure everyday. Don't give up because you can do it!

15 Simple Ways To Lower Your Blood Pressure Naturally After 40 Without Complicated Diets

Table of Contents

15 Simple Ways To Lower Your Blood Pressure Naturally After 40 Without Complicated Diets

15 Simple Ways To Lower Your Blood Pressure Naturally After 40 Without Complicated Diets

Introduction

High blood pressure or hypertension is a common and dangerous disease in America and the whole world. According to the Center for Disease Control and Prevention (CDC) about one out of every three Americans has hypertension or high blood pressure and the World Health Organization (WHO) stated that in 2014 about 22% of all adults in the world18 years and over had high blood pressure.

According to the CDC, hypertension increases the risk of heart disease and stroke which are among the leading causes of death in America. It may also lead to other complications like kidney failure and blindness. One of the most frustrating aspects of having high blood pressure is that most people quickly give up on lifestyle changes and rely only on medications to manage it.

15 Simple Ways To Lower Your Blood Pressure Naturally After 40 Without Complicated Diets

A lot of people want to take steps on their own to lower their blood pressure but find the available options too complicated to follow. The reasons why people want to take action on their own range from a desire to have more control over their health or wellness, to a fear of potential side effects from conventional medications. A third and very important reason is that research has shown that some simple natural steps can actually lower one's blood pressure. You can lower your blood pressure naturally by making certain changes to your lifestyle, Right Now!

The most effective ways involve making small but significant changes to various aspects of our daily lives. These will involve how we relate to one another, how we eat, and how we try to make our dreams come true.

15 Simple Ways To Lower Your Blood Pressure Naturally After 40 Without Complicated Diets

This book will show you easy steps you can take to naturally help reduce your blood pressure without relying on complicated diets. The first step in this process is getting a better understanding of yourself. This is the first step in the Compass Method.

If you find and use natural ways to reduce your blood pressure, you will end up needing fewer medications. The fewer medications you take, the lower the number of side effects, you have to deal with in your life. The more you reduce your blood pressure, the more you reduce your chances of having high blood pressure-related complications. The fewer complications you have, the more time you will have to enjoy yourself now and in your golden years!!!

15 Simple Ways To Lower Your Blood Pressure Naturally After 40 Without Complicated Diets

What you need to know about your blood pressure

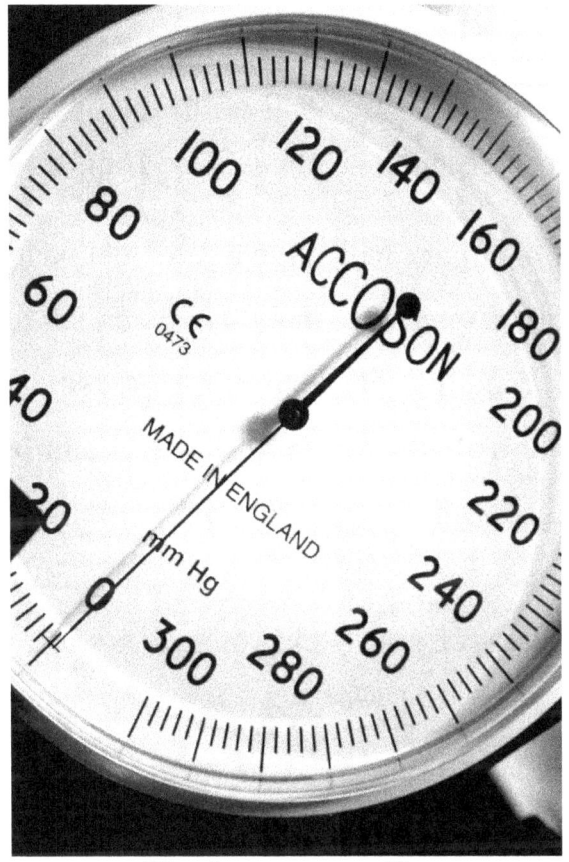

Blood pressure cuff

The **normal blood pressure** is less than **120/80 mmHg**. A systolic blood pressure or upper reading between **120 -139 mmHg** is **pre-hypertension**, while the second number or the diastolic pressure lies between **80 and 89 mmHg. Stage 1 hypertension** = systolic140 **to 159 mmHg** and diastolic of **90 to 99mmhg. Stage 2 hypertension** will be systolic or first readings of **160 mmHg or higher** and diastolic will be **100mmHg or more.**

This figure will serve as a guideline to the levels of blood pressure and their potential for damage to the body. **Hypertension is usually treated or controlled through a combination of medications or lifestyle changes or natural means**. When this is not done, damage to heart, heart disease, and other health problems like stroke, kidney disease and loss of vision will occur. Repeated brain damage from strokes can lead to dementia or Alzheimer-like symptoms. Severe hypertension can lead to blindness.

The good news is that if you take action today, you will give yourself a good chance of avoiding these complications. Sadly according to the CDC about 52% of the 70 million people who have high blood pressure do not have it under control.

The CDC also states that about 50% of the people who have their first heart attack and about two out of three people who have their first stoke already have a blood pressure of more than 160/95 mmHg or stage 2 hypertension.

Blood Pressure	mmHg
Normal	SBP<120, DBP<80
Prehypertension	SBP 120-139,DBP 80-89
Stage 1 hypertension	SBP140-159,DBP 90-99
Stage 2 hypertension	SBP 160 or more, DBP100 or more

SBP=Systolic Blood Pressure

DBP=Diastolic Blood Pressure; mmHg = millimeters of Mercury

These sad outcomes occur because people take their health for granted. Don't take your health for granted. Check your blood pressure today. High blood pressure is mostly symptomless and you will not know you have it unless you know your numbers. You can check your blood pressure either with your doctor, at your local pharmacy or at home with your own blood pressure device.

According to the Mayo Clinic, hypertension can be broadly divided into **primary or secondary hypertension**. About 95% of the cases of hypertension are due to essential or primary hypertension and is usually without symptoms. The remaining 5% of cases are due to secondary hypertension. The causes of secondary hypertension include:

Thyroid problems

Defects in blood vessels

Pregnancy problems

Kidney problems

Adrenal gland tumors

Obstructive sleep apnea (Sleep problems)

Medications like birth control pills, cold remedies and some prescriptions

Drug misuse-cocaine and amphetamine

Alcohol misuse or abuse

Other forms of hypertension include **isolated systolic hypertension, white coat hypertension and malignant or accelerated hypertension**. White coat hypertension occurs when blood pressure goes up in clinics or when blood pressure is taken by healthcare professionals and is usually related to anxiety. If it persists it needs to be treated. Isolated systolic high blood pressure occurs when the top number remains above

140mmHg but the bottom one is almost less than 90 mmHg. According to the CDC the classification of hypertension is determined by which number is higher when both numbers fall into different categories.

According to the National Institutes of Health (NIH), **malignant or accelerated hypertension** is very high blood pressure that rises suddenly and is associated with a diastolic blood pressure that is often 130 mmHg or more. It affects about 1% of people with high blood pressure and is common in children, young adults and African-Americans. **It is a life-threatening emergency** condition often associated with the following:

Brain damage (stroke, seizures)

Blindness

Renal Failure (Kidney Failure)

Lung damage (Fluid in lungs)

Heart damage (heart attack, heart failure, pain and heart rhythm problems).

ACTION TIP

CHECK YOUR BLOOD PRESSURE TODAY

15 Simple Ways To Lower Your Blood Pressure Naturally After 40 Without Complicated Diets

The Compass Method For Reducing Blood Pressure

The key to avoiding or reducing your chances of having some of these complications or health problems associated with high blood pressure is to check your blood pressure daily, take your medications and make lifestyle adjustments or changes. The Compass Method shows you simple steps you can consistently take to make the lifestyle adjustments that will help you reduce your blood pressure and dependence on medications. In order to do this you have to change your mind-set and be prepared to take effective daily action, instead of continually looking for a single magical solution or a silver bullet.

Even in nature, it is self-evident that simple solutions are the most enduring. They are easy to learn, fun to do and lead to more consistent results.

.

This is why the Compass Method for reducing blood pressure is based on the following simple steps.

1, Know yourself better.

This will help your adjust your mindset, expectations and build on your strengths.

2, Reduce stress

It is easy to simply say "reduce stress" without giving details about how to overcome chronic stress that may arise out of your daily pressure points. You will learn about how to do this in this book.

3, Improve your daily emotional well being

4, Lose weight

5, Adjust your diet

6, Maintain Balance

7, Quit smoking

8, **Manage your finances**

9, Take daily action

10, Review, Adjust and Persist (RAP)

Make your own version of the Compass Method sustainable through individualized adjustments.

15 Simple Ways To Lower Your Blood Pressure Naturally After 40 Without Complicated Diets

Know yourself: How to use the compass health profiles to know yourself better

The compass health profiles are the foundation for the compass method for transformational living. You can apply the method to your blood pressure and reduce it. Here are the components of the compass profile.

Compass Health Profiles:

C = Community Relationships.

O = Operational capacity profile.

M= Metabolic profile.

P= Physical profile.

A= Ambition profile.

S= Spiritual profile.

S = Self Knowledge profile.

15 Simple Ways To Lower Your Blood Pressure Naturally After 40 Without Complicated Diets

How do you use these profiles to help you live a healthier and happier life? According to current medical research those who have good **community relationships** with themselves, their family and their friends tend to live longer and healthier lives.

When was the last time you said, "I love you" to your spouse or lover? When was the last time you called your brother or sister? When was the last time you forgave yourself? When was the last time you shared a joke with your co-worker? What if you are from a dysfunctional family? What if you are not even on talking terms with your brothers and sisters? Don't sweat it. Just make a phone call or send a text message. Why? It will help you reduce stress and have more energy for all the fun things you would like to do with your life. Nothing in life is perfect, so if you find some of these steps too hard to take, begin with the actions you can take today. Stop blaming yourself for everything.

15 Simple Ways To Lower Your Blood Pressure Naturally After 40 Without Complicated Diets

Answering or asking these questions will help you recognize your own relationship stress triggers or pressure points. It will help you understand yourself better and become a better manager of the conflict that inevitably occurs within different types of relationships. Just remember that you can also make your friends part of your family. After all, good companionship from those we live with and interact with everyday helps us live longer and better.

I don't really want to make things more complicated than they need to be. Basically through your **operational capacity profile,** you ask yourself how you get things done and how you can improve. The simplest way to do this is to look back at your life and find out which method of preparation and execution has worked the best for you in your most successful projects.

15 Simple Ways To Lower Your Blood Pressure Naturally After 40 Without Complicated Diets

Include in your projects things like getting ready for Christmas and Thanksgiving or getting ready for a wedding or tasks as simple as going to work on time and cleaning your house. For most people, the best way to tackle most projects is to start on time and break them down into small simple steps. For others every project is eventually done at the last minute.

If you like to get things done at the last minute, it means you tend to procrastinate and underestimate how much time you need to get things to done. Remember that inadequate preparation leads to failure. To reduce your blood pressure naturally you will have to start with a small plan and build on it slowly, in a way that suits your internal and external circumstances.

Your **Metabolic profile** will include both your nutritional and metabolic analysis. You get your metabolic analysis by getting your physiological and laboratory tests done. This will include your blood pressure, cholesterol level and other metabolic tests your doctor deems necessary. Of course getting these results will make it easy for you to know which aspect of your health profile you need to focus on improving.

Take action today, measure your blood pressure today, even if you feel you are in excellent health. This was precisely what happened to my friend, Philip, who thought he had excellent health until a pharmacy blood pressure checkup showed his blood pressure was 160 mmHg over110 mmHg. This result startled him and he went to see his doctor the very next day. This is what I call putting your metabolic profile to good use. Do you know your Metabolic Profile?

The Physical Profile includes your weight, height, waist circumference and BMI. It also includes your heart rate and lung function. These factors are important because it is important to know your health status before you can engage in vigorous exercise. The main exercise protocol proposed in **the Compass Method** is mild to moderate activities like **walking**, dancing, jump ropes and pushups. Those who are more used to vigorous exercise like playing basketball, tennis, baseball need to remember to check with their doctor that they are healthy enough to continue to exercise vigorously as they get older. One advantage of staying physically active is that it helps us burn off excessive energy that would have been converted to fat that ultimately clog our arteries.

The Ambition profile looks at your job and finances and satisfaction with your life. This is important because without good finances or insurance it is much more difficult to take good care of your health. I know most health books do not include this profile but the Ambition profile measures your ability to get things done or to make adjustments when they are required. Set measurable goals like reducing your weight by 5Lbs or your blood pressure by 5mmHg.

The remaining two profiles are **Spirituality and Self Knowledge**, both of which examine your psychospiritual makeup. They will help you have a better understanding of your personality, character and connection with God and the universe. A better understanding of your psychological strengths and weaknesses will help you know your limitations, when it comes to choosing pathways to better health. It will also help you to anticipate problems, quarrels and pressure points. On the spiritual side of the equation, more and more studies are beginning to show that those who meditate or are truly prayerful are better able to handle health challenges than those who do neither. Of course I realize that there are different interpretations of what it means to be spiritual and that one size does not fit all.

ACTION TIP

UNDERSTAND YOURSELF BETTER

.

.

Know yourself: know your passion

Knowing your passion is part of how you know yourself. This is because unless you have a better understanding of yourself, you will always stumble or have difficulty as you try to relate to others and to yourself. Your passion is part of what connects you to the world. What one thing or item would you like to change in the world? Your answer here could be a multitude of things including providing better drinking water, helping underprivileged children or to help stop an animal from becoming extinct.

What do you do in your spare time? You probably spend time developing one of your hobbies or talents. You may spend time hiking, writing, playing music, exercising or doing whatever you enjoy.

15 Simple Ways To Lower Your Blood Pressure Naturally After 40 Without Complicated Diets

What makes you smile? All those things that make you smile are things that you love and enjoy doing. Of course, it doesn't have to be an item. Spending time with your grandchildren or visiting a senior home can be other things that put a smile on your face.

Go through this list and start writing down your answers. From here you want to see if there is one thing that gets repeated again and again. If so, chances are that this is your passion.

By finding your passion and making it a greater part of your life, you will enjoy more of your daily activities and cut down on stress. This will help you reduce your blood pressure. The good thing about being over 40 years of age is that you have had plenty of time to discover a lot about yourself. This means you probably have a good idea about your strengths and weaknesses. Focus more on your strengths and take daily action to enjoy your hobbies and interests. Take action that will help your talents and gifts flourish instead worrying about your weaknesses and what negative people have to say about you.

The more you focus on the positive, the less stressed out you will be. The lower your blood pressure will become.

ACTION TIP

KNOW YOUR PASSION

15 Simple Ways To Lower Your Blood Pressure Naturally After 40 Without Complicated Diets

How to adjust your diet and reduce your blood pressure

The problem most people have is that they get so caught up with trying new ways of eating healthy that they keep on changing plans. This is like trying to build a house without ever getting past the design or plan.

If you really want to lower your blood pressure through healthy eating, you have to find a simple plan and stick to it. You have to find healthy foods you like and stick to them .For example, celery can help lower blood pressure, but you can only get the full benefit if you consistently eat it day in day out.

Instead of chasing the latest complicated diet, adjust what you eat everyday to what fits your budget and is enjoyable for you. This is part of the compass method, because we believe it will be easier to make adjustments to the food you are used to eating than to try to acquire a new taste. Most people that begin a new diet find it hard to sustain and end up quitting before they can see tangible results.

One way to adjust your diet is to find a way to eat right within your culture. This means finding ways to make adjustments to eating habits that you grew up with, without going crazy by trying to count calories. This is a simple but effective approach to eating right in a culturally sensitive way. Different cultures have their dominant food types and specialties which the population of the culture eats regularly.

The dominant or staple food in Asia is rice. In Africa people eat a lot of "fufu" or pounded food like cassava and yams. In Italy it is pasta, in America people eat a lot of pizza and other fast food like hamburgers, fried chicken and French fries.

15 Simple Ways To Lower Your Blood Pressure Naturally After 40 Without Complicated Diets

The first step to take would be to cut down the servings or portions of your regular meal by half. For this example let us use about half or a third to reduce your energy intake. You fill the gap with vegetables and fruits. If you feel pangs of hunger, snack with nuts, drink plenty of water or take some fruits. Please do not take soda for water.

The more your servings are reduced, the more weight you would lose. This makes sense since less food intake means less energy intake. The short fall in energy will be obtained from excess body fat resulting in weight loss. However, reduced servings may mean more hunger pangs. To deal with this, eat more fruits, vegetables and fibers as fillers. Fibers are especially good for your system because they help to increase bowel movement. This has the added effect of making your digestive system more efficient.

15 Simple Ways To Lower Your Blood Pressure Naturally After 40 Without Complicated Diets

Eating food rich in fruits and whole grains helps to lower your blood pressure. Do you know by how much? It is by about 13mmHg. Of course this will also include reducing the intake of saturated fat and cholesterol. Whole grains contain a lot of fiber. Foods like brown rice, oat meal, millet and barley are whole grains.

For different cultures and settings, different modifications to familiar eating habits can be made. In America this would entail cutting down on fast foods, soda and other processed foods. You can do this by going to eat fast food only once a month. If you cannot do this, start by either eating only small sizes or eating only half of their sandwich.

For the good of your own health, do not go along with food choices that will not be good for your health just because people from your culture may challenge you or make fun of you. Your culture is supposed to help you, not to kill you. You can do this by finding a way to eat right within your culture.

Before you make the final decision on the adjustments to make to your food, do a 72 hour food audit. You can do this by simply writing down the food, drinks and snacks you have eaten in the past 72 hours. When I did my audit I found out that while my goal was to reduce sodium intake to about 1500 mg per day, I was eating about 10 slices of bread everyday. This meant I was already getting too much sodium just from bread alone without even adding my other sources of sodium. On the average a slide of bread contains 150 mg of sodium.

My initial approach was to simply cut down my slices of bread to 5 instead of 10. I found it difficult to do this because I did not want to address the reason why I ate a lot of bread. The reason was that I wanted to have a sense of "fullness' after every meal. To tackle this craving, I had to start drinking more water with each meal.

I started by drinking a glass of water before each meal. This helped me feel full, without eating as much as before. After a while, I was able to consistently cut down my slices of bread to 2 to 4, instead of 10. As a result my sodium intake also reduced. **This was an example of the Compass method in action.**

The good news is that this approach is not unique to me. You too can do this. Research has shown that drinking water before a meal will help to expand your stomach. This approach will make you feel full when you are actually 80% full. This is important because eating only up to 80 % full was one of the common practices of people of

Okinawa in Japan, who have the highest number of centenarians in the world. My suggestion is that you drink at least two glasses of water per meal.

The other good tips which came from my food audit were that, I ate too much beef and rice, with little or no fruits and vegetables. I also found out I ate too much white bread and butter. I switched to whole wheat bread, which contains much more fiber than white bread and I stopped adding butter to my bread. In addition, instead of eating just white rice, I started eating brown rice. Brown rice has more fiber and more energy.

To increase my intake of fruits and vegetables, I started eating every rice meal with salads consisting of cabbage, carrots, broccoli, spinach and bananas. Eating a colorful variety of fruits and vegetables per meal made my meal more healthy. I am sure that if you do same, your meals will become more healthy and full of antioxidants. Antioxidants help our bodies to remove or counter the effects of free radicals that can damage our bodies.

Whatever you discover, start small. Remember that little drops of water make the mighty ocean. This thought will help you, even when you feel overwhelmed by the thought of changing your eating habits. When I changed my eating habits, I started by making small changes like adding salads to every meal of rice that I had. I found the whole idea difficult initially but I had to remind myself that I did not want to spend my golden years, chronically ill and being moved from one nursing home or hospital to another. I took time to find the combination   of fruits and vegetables that worked best for me. Try a few combinations to find out what will work best for you.

15 Simple Ways To Lower Your Blood Pressure Naturally After 40 Without Complicated Diets

Once you begin to add fruits, vegetables and other food varieties make sure you make enough adjustments to make your meals healthy.

DO VAMB

Variety-Do not eat the same meal day in day out. Why? It gets boring after a while and you will soon find yourself looking less forward to eating healthy.

Adequacy- Provide sufficient essential nutrients. Make sure your food contains adequate but moderate portions of fat, proteins, carbohydrates and vitamins. Eat enough food to fill full, when you eat. If you don't fill full after a meal you will find yourself eating too much sugary snacks in between meals to get more energy.

Moderation- Do not eat a particular food too much just because you like it. This was like how I used to a lot of white bread and soda just because, I liked them. Concentrate on eating non-processed food instead of on processed food like bacon and "ready –to-go" meals like frozen burritos and pizzas. They are convenient but have high sugar and sodium content! Eating fruits and vegetables is one way to increase the intake of potassium which helps to counter the effects of sodium on the blood pressure.

Balance-Do not let a food type dominate your meals,-too much beef or bread. When you do your own food audit, you will know what food dominates your eating pattern and what adjustments you need to make. When I did my food audit, I found out that my eating pattern was dominated by rice and bread. I made changes. I added more, corn, fruits and nuts to my daily food.

Be particularly careful with how much soda or beer you drink. Beer has a lot of calories with little ingredients. Drinking too much beer may cost you some important vitamins like vitamin B6. Another way balance your meal would be to halve your intake of all pure or added fats.

You need to be careful when you start cutting down carbohydrate like white bread, white rice or pasta. This will make you lose weight quickly because it is usually stored in the body as glycogen which contains water. You need to be careful because the brain gets most of its energy from glucose and if it does not get enough you begin to feel tired, weak, unable to sleep and ill. Unless you switch to fiber-rich carbohydrate sources like baked sweet potato, whole grain bread, barley, oat meal and brown rice, you may end up quitting after a few weeks. This is why **the compass method is** about adjustments and individualized modifications.

To make your meals healthier eat chicken, fish, beans, cottage cheese, or low fat yogurt. Have eggs, nuts and red meat occasionally but not every day. When you eat chicken or turkey, eat skinless since most of the fat contained in this type of meat is contained within the skin. Grilling is better than frying, and always aim to use unsaturated oils like corn, and olive oils for cooking. Reduce the fat content in your milk products. If you are currently drinking whole milk, reduce to 2% fat; from 2% reduce to 1%. Choose lower-fat cheese and yogurt. When you buy yogurt, also check that it does not contain sugar. The good thing about reducing to 1% fat milk is that it remains tasteful.

Plan your meals and snacks ahead of time. Take time to plan at least one lunch and dinner every week without meat or cheese. Build those meals around whole grains, vegetables and beans to increase fiber and reduce fat. If you want to have something to chew on, get some fish or tofu. You can make every Friday your fish meal day. One quick plan I have for snacks is a combination of unsalted peanuts, bananas and dark chocolate. It makes me fill full and it helps to reduce blood pressure. Try it and give me a feedback.

Have at least five servings of fruit every day. This can be for dessert or snacks. Choose fruit that is in season. One fruit, I like a lot is apple. My rule is to take an apple per meal. If you can, go for those red delicious apples because they contain pectin, a fiber that helps to promote healthy cholesterol levels and contain more amounts of antioxidants than many other types of apples.

15 Simple Ways To Lower Your Blood Pressure Naturally After 40 Without Complicated Diets

Drink water instead of sodas, juices, milky drinks or alcohol. Avoid diet soda - the sweet taste only encourages you to crave sugar. Hot water with a slice of lemon can be very refreshing in the morning. Aim to drink about eight glasses of water everyday.

ACTION TIPS

ADJUST YOUR DAILY FOOD

DO A 72-HOUR FOOD AUDIT

CUT DOWN YOUR SERVING PORTIONS

EAT FOOD RICH IN FRUITS AND WHOLE GRAINS

MODIFY YOUR TYPICAL CULTURAL FOOD

DRINK TWO GLASSES OF WATER BEFORE EVERY MEAL

BALANCE YOUR DAILY FOOD TYPES

PLAN FOR YOUR SNACKS

CUT DOWN ON SODA AND SNACKS

15 Simple Ways To Lower Your Blood Pressure Naturally After 40 Without Complicated Diets

Adjust your diet: Reduce sodium intake

When most people that are hypertensive think of reducing sodium, they end up doing only one thing, they stop adding sodium to the food they eat. They then complain that though they have stopped adding salt to their food, their blood pressure has remained high. This is usually disappointing because the food has become less tasteful, yet the desired effect of a reduced blood pressure has not been achieved.

This usually happens because other sources of sodium have not been accounted for. This includes salt used in cooking and salt used in preserving pre-cooked food. The first is obvious while the second will involve some research. Do you know how much salt is contained in pre-cooked burrito, pizza or hotdog? All three contain significant amounts of hidden salt, which we need to identify or eliminate to reduce our total daily intake of salt or sodium. On average one burrito has 470mg to 1200mg of sodium and one slice of pizza contains about 190 mg to 900 mg of sodium. Pizza with vegetable toppings and less cheese has less sodium. One average hot dog has about 470 mg of sodium. These are huge numbers if you are trying to keep your daily sodium intake to 1500mg of sodium or less. This is one of the reasons why cutting down on fast foods or completely eliminating them is strongly recommended.

Adding spices to your food instead of salt can make your food more tasty without increasing your sodium intake. After a period of adjustment this becomes second nature and one of the benefits of reduced sodium or salt intake is lowered blood pressure.

15 Simple Ways To Lower Your Blood Pressure Naturally After 40 Without Complicated Diets

If you are over 40 and you want to cut down on sodium so that you can reduce your blood pressure then you have to **learn to read your nutrition facts.** The nutrition facts are labels on foods that explain the nutrients or ingredients they contain.

Generally, when I look at my nutrition facts, I also look at my sodium, fiber, and fat content. I know people sometimes ignore their sodium content, thinking it does not really matter. Well, it does. When comparing a loaf of bread with a can of soda, you will find that a single serving of bread contains 150 milligrams of sodium, while the can of soda contains 65 milligrams of sodium per serving size. Can you believe it?

Did you know that we only need about 2300 milligrams of salt everyday? This is equivalent to one flat teaspoon of salt. If you make it a habit to read the nutritional facts on your food label you will not only learn about the ingredients in your food but you will also learn how to limit your sodium intake to about 2300mg or less a day. As a known hypertensive or a person with additional risk factors for heart disease, you need to aim for 1500 mg per day.

This means that if you are over 40 and a hypertensive, your goal should be to eat less than 1500mg of sodium per day. The good thing to remember is that reducing sodium intake can lower your blood pressure by about 5mmHg. Now if you intend to eat about 1500 milligrams of sodium per day, and start your day with ten slices of bread, you have just eaten 1500 milligrams of sodium to start your day. Then any other sodium you eat for the rest of day will be in excess of your target.

15 Simple Ways To Lower Your Blood Pressure Naturally After 40 Without Complicated Diets

If you enjoy eating bread because of its fibers you may unwittingly be eating too much sodium. Failing to read or use your nutritional facts is like going to a fancy restaurant and ordering your food without reading the menu? How will you know if the food you are ordering is what you like or what you will enjoy eating? Food with 140mg or less of sodium preserving has low sodium, 35mg of sodium or less per serving has very low sodium, 5 mg of sodium per serving is considered sodium free.

By reading your food facts you will know how much sodium each choice you make will add to daily intake of sodium. This is type of knowledge will ultimately help you to control your sodium intake and reduce your pressure without putting too much effort into it. After all, knowledge is power. The more you know about the daily factors that can affect your health, and take action, the more empowered you shall become!

ACTION TIPS

READ NUTRITION FACTS
REDUCE SODIUM INTAKE

Adjust your diet: Eat your food slowly

Even if you did all the modifications to make your daily meals healthy but ended up eating fast, you will end up over eating. Eat slowly. The body is slow to register when you are full and it is easy to eat too much if you are racing through your meals. You can easily do this if you eat and do other things at the same time.

Here are a number of ways people eat and do other activities at the same time that could make them not eat slowly:

Eating and watching TV. If you eat and watch TV you do not pay as much attention as you should to your food so you end up eating fast and shoveling your food down your throat. Try as much as you can to switch off the TV when you eat. That includes snacks as well as meals. Studies have proved that we eat larger portions in front of the TV, probably because we are much less aware of what we are eating.

Driving and eating. Most people do this, especially after buying fast food. However it is difficult to eat slowly, when you are concentrating both on eating and following your driving directions. What invariably happens is that we gobble our food with little or no chewing.

Talking and eating on the phone will make you eat your food fast. This too, is an avoidable distraction that helps to reduce your concentration on the actual chewing and eating of food.

Eating and working is another habit that makes you eat your food in a hurry instead of slowly.

15 Simple Ways To Lower Your Blood Pressure Naturally After 40 Without Complicated Diets

This is a very common practice among handy men. They pick up their hamburgers and chew on them while they hammer nails into the wall. Two problems here are poor digestion and more accidents or injuries. Give one activity your full attention, then move on to the next.

Choose food that you can chew. Again this will increase your fiber intake, and the act of chewing will make you feel more satisfied too. This means eating fruit instead of drinking juice. If you have soup, make sure it is chunky.

Another way you can get yourself to eat more slowly and enjoy your food more is to find a place where you eat on a regular basis everyday. This could be eating breakfast at home, instead of in your car. If due to your busy schedule you cannot do this in the morning then make it your super. Instead of sitting in front of the TV after work

,eating and watching TV, sit at your dining table and eat your super slowly.

If you follow these tips regularly, you will find that the portion of food you will end up eating will be greatly decreased and you will enjoy your food more. The overall effect will be that you will lose weight and reduce your blood pressure precipitously.

ACTION TIP

FOCUS ON EATING AND EAT SLOWLY

Adjust your diet: Super foods you can use to reduce your blood pressure

You can reduce your blood pressure or chances of having a heart attack through the use of super foods like olives, pomegranate, yoghurt or dark chocolate. A study done by the American Academy of Neurology found that olives and olive oil can lower blood pressure and cholesterol levels. Interestingly, lowering both blood pressure and cholesterol, reduces the important risk factors for heart attacks.

Olive oil can be used regularly for cooking or for salad dressing. This will mean spending more on oil since olive oil costs more than the regular oil. Spending more on super foods like olive that will help to lower blood pressure is probably better than spending money on fast food and alcohol.

15 Simple Ways To Lower Your Blood Pressure Naturally After 40 Without Complicated Diets

Pomegranates can also help you to keep the heart healthy. One, it has a lot of antioxidants, two, it can help lower the blood pressure. A British study found that drinking a glass of pomegranates daily can help to lower blood pressure. Make sure you drink 100% juice, not just mixtures and other drinks that contain minimal extracts of pomegranate.

Eating yogurts frequently can also help to lower your blood pressure. This does not necessarily mean eating yogurts every day.

Dark chocolate is another food that can lower blood pressure. Eat dark chocolate with at least 70% cocoa. It might be a little a bit bitter but after a while you will get used to it.

Celery is a crunchy vegetable that contains a compound called 3-n-butyl phthalide that relaxes the smooth muscle lining in blood vessels, reducing blood pressure. Some studies have found that eating about 4 ribs of celery a day can lower blood pressure by about by 12 to 14 percent. One stalk of celery contains 312 mg of potassium.

Garlic has anti-inflammatory and antiviral properties that can fight coronary heart disease by unplugging arteries. The gas that garlic produces in the stomach relaxes your arteries and lowers blood pressure. Eating garlic regularly can help to reduce your blood pressure.

Bananas have a high content of potassium, which is known to lower blood pressure and reduce the risk of stroke. Bananas are also low in sodium. Just three large bananas per meal can provide an accumulated total daily dose of potassium that will help to reduce blood pressure and fend off various cardiovascular diseases. According the Colorado State University (CSU) the aim should be to eat about 4,700 mg of potassium (K^+) per day which is equivalent to Adequate Intake of potassium for a day. One medium sized banana has 422 mg of potassium. If you find eating three large bananas per meal too boring, use variety to achieve the same goals. Eat celery, bananas, carrots and oranges which contain a lot of potassium.

Tomatoes contain lycopene, an antioxidant that helps protect your cells from the damaging effects of free radicals. The lycopene and other carotenoids found in tomatoes help in reducing high blood pressure and lowering the risk of heart disease. According to the American Heart Journal eating about 250mg of tomato extract for eight weeks can significantly lower both systolic and diastolic blood pressure among those who have high blood pressure. According the Colorado State University (CSU) on potassium in fruits and vegetables, one large tomato contains 300 mg of potassium.

ACTION TIPS

COOK WITH OLIVE OIL

EAT POMEGRANATES

EAT YOGURTS AND DARK CHOCOLATE

EAT BANANA AND CELERY

EAT TOMATOES

15 Simple Ways To Lower Your Blood Pressure Naturally After 40 Without Complicated Diets

Reduce stress: reduce your risk of a heart attack

As a hypertensive you may have heard it said to you on more than one occasion that reducing stress is very important. Everybody talks about reducing stress through mediation and spirituality, but few people focus on how to deal with or reduce day by day stress. Yet it is the chronicity of daily stress that makes it deadly. This is especially true for those with hypertension who already have a heart carrying the burden of pumping blood under tremendous pressure. This has a huge chance of a breakdown in the form of heart attack.

How can you reduce your chances of having a heart attack as a hypertensive? First, check your blood pressure regularly. Take your medications and visit your doctor regularly. In addition to doing all of the above, also empower yourself by getting more information and getting more answers.

Would you not like to know what is your likelihood of having a heart attack in the next 10 years? I would want to know because heart disease is among the leading cause of death for those over 40 in most parts of the world, including the United States and Western Europe.

The problem is that most of us still feel that heart attacks are things that happen to others. We do not feel it will happen to us, so we take little or no precautions to modify our risks for such adverse health events. While for others with normal health status, this might be a minimal risk for those over 40, age compounds the problem.

Factors that are used to calculate your cardiovascular risk factor include:

*Age

15 Simple Ways To Lower Your Blood Pressure Naturally After 40 Without Complicated Diets

*Sex

*Race

*Family history of heart disease or diabetes

*Lipid profile as stated above.

*BMI

*Personality type

Age, sex and race are factors that cannot usually be changed, but you can use them to calculate your cardiovascular risk points and then convert the points to percentage risk for heart attack over a 10-year period.

Knowing your lipid profile is important because you can use it in computing your cardiovascular risk. Your lipid profile, includes, your triglyceride level, total cholesterol, HDL (High Density Lipoprotein) or good cholesterol, and LDL (Low density Lipoprotein) or bad cholesterol.

15 Simple Ways To Lower Your Blood Pressure Naturally After 40 Without Complicated Diets

Here is an example of the cardiovascular points for a 45- year-old- man Joseph with a low HDL (<35) and a total cholesterol of 220 and a blood pressure of 130/80 mmHg, who is not diabetic but smokes. Being a 45 year old male, would give him 6 points, If he was a woman the points would be 5. A HDL of less than 35 would give him 2 points. Total cholesterol of 220 would be equivalent to 2 points. Smoking would give him 4 points, while a blood pressure of 130/80mmHg is equivalent to 3 points.

This calculation means Joseph has (6+2+2+4+3)=17 points and would translate to at least 29.4% risk of cardiovascular disease(CVD) in 10 years .What does this mean?

According to the Framingham Heart Study, moderate risk ,is a 10 year CVD risk of less than 10%,moderately high risk is 10-20% and high risk is 20%and above. This means that Joseph has a high risk for cardiovascular disease. For Joseph, the man in this example, his numbers mean that 29 out of 100 people with his risk profile will have a heart attack in the next 10 years This is too high a risk as confirmed by the Framingham Heart Study.

The advantage of finding out your risk factor before having a heart attack is that it gives you an opportunity to take action. For, Joseph he can change his risk for a heart disease by quitting smoking, this will take away,4 points from his 17. Making his HDL 50 and his total cholesterol less than 160, would give him points of (-1),and (0).This means his new total CVD points will be (6+(-1)+0+0+3)=8, which will be equivalent to 6.7%,10 year risk of CVD.

The other important ratio that is worth calculating is the ratio between your triglycerides and your total low density lipoprotein (LDL).

15 Simple Ways To Lower Your Blood Pressure Naturally After 40 Without Complicated Diets

Essentially this means that by taking action and modifying his risk factors through eating healthy and quitting smoking, Joseph reduced his risk of having a heart attack by more than half. He changed his risk of a heart attack from 29 out of 100 people in 10 years to 7 out of 100 people in 10 years, for people with a similar heart risk profile.

There is a difference between knowing what to do, and doing it. Through the Compass Method, I will continue to share with you the different strategies you can use to reduce the risk of heart disease. The first step would be to help you get a better understanding of yourself, then help you increase physical activity, sleep better, reduce stress and eat more fruits and vegetables. I am certainly looking forward to sharing more details with you as you continue to read this book on the simple and fast ways you can develop a personalized blueprint that will help you reduce your blood pressure naturally.

ACTION TIPS

MANAGE YOUR CONVERSATIONS

EXERCISE EVERYDAY

SLEEP WELL

IMPROVE YOUR EMOTIONAL WELL-BEING

QUIT SMOKING

Reduce stress: Manage your Conversations

Your daily conversations are an important part of your daily life. It is through them that you relate to people in your community either at work, at home or at other social gatherings. If you have hypertension or high blood pressure you are probably familiar with the idea of watching what you eat by not adding salt to your food or meals and cutting down on your weight. **However have you ever considered that you can also manage your blood pressure through your conversations with others?** You can do this by using some of the strategies I shall share with you on how to cope with the stress that can arise through your daily conversations.

Coping with our conversations is important because this is an activity we all participate in everyday. We interact with others through our conversations. We do this by listening to others, talking to others and responding to what others say or have failed to say or do. Unless we are able to make the distinction between what needs a response what does not, we may end up getting worked up. The idea of getting worked up is even a less acceptable option for you when you have high blood pressure.

A simple strategy for coping with the potential emotional tension that may sometimes arise from our daily conversations would be divide our conversations or activities into 'Little rocks" and "heavy rocks". Little rocks are those conversations you can either afford to overlook or can decide to ignore without losing out significantly. What is an example of little rock conversation? If you are in the midst of a conversation with your brother and he is arguing that the sun goes round the earth, what will you say? Will you continue to argue even when you have shown him irrevocable evidence and he continues to argue? Arguing for arguing sake will only get you worked up and build up your blood pressure. This is an example of the "Little rocks" in a conversation. Let it go! **You don't have to have the last word.**

You have more important things to do with your time and energy. Spending quality time with your family should be considered a 'big rock". You could go and watch a movie with your wife or partner. You could go swimming or go for a walk in the park. You could spend more time with your family and friends.

ACTION TIPS

FOCUS ON THE BIG ROCKS
YOU DON'T HAVE TO HAVE THE LAST WORD

15 Simple Ways To Lower Your Blood Pressure Naturally After 40 Without Complicated Diets

Reduce stress: Exercise everyday

Participating in daily exercise will make you healthier and also diminish the effects of stress on your body. We know that chronic stress can lead to increased high blood pressure, increased plaques in blood vessels and increased stress hormones.

To help increase your immune system and decrease your stress level, exercise everyday. This can be as simple as walking everyday or as sophisticated as doing yoga at home daily.

Walking shoes are great because they make walking more comfortable. However do not use their absence as an excuse for not doing your daily exercise if you are committed to one.

15 Simple Ways To Lower Your Blood Pressure Naturally After 40 Without Complicated Diets

As you go through your daily activities, make it a point to walk a little further. One of my favorite tricks for doing this is to park far away from the entrance each time I go to the grocery store or the mall. This will help you take a few more steps everyday. Try it. You will be surprised how effective this can become for you without changing your lifestyle a great deal.

There are several different exercises that you can do to help eliminate the stress in your life. Walking is among the best, as you can easily lose yourself and your troubles by walking. Even if it is just around the block, walking can do wonders for your health. It can also help to reduce your stress level.

If you have a lot of stress in your life, you may want to consider a gym. Working out and then sitting in the sauna is also a good way to relieve tension. If your gym has a pool, you may find swimming to be very beneficial as well, as it helps you to relax.

If you do not like walking or going to the gym, consider going for swimming exercises, joining a dance class or even playing tennis. If you find yourself doing a lot of standing or sitting as part of your job or daily life, consider bending down to pick something up without using a pick up stick or moving the item towards you with your foot when standing.

The bottom line is that if you find any exercise pattern that fits into your life style and do it regularly, you will see that daily stress in your life will reduce. The other benefit of daily exercise is that it can help you reduce your blood pressure. Consistently doing exercise everyday can help you lower your blood pressure. However, if you begin then stop, you will lose the health benefits associated with exercise.

I am not saying become a weekend warrior and put yourself into an exercise regimen you can barely cope with. Start with increasing your daily physical activity like mowing your lawn, cleaning your house, washing your car and going for daily walks. Aim for a combined total of about 45 minutes of physical activity most days of the week.

This will help to reduce your blood pressure because exercise makes the heart a better pump so that more volume of blood is pumped per heart beat with less expenditure of energy. This is because the pressure in the arteries is reduced so that the force required to pump blood is also reduced. Hence the reduction in blood pressure.

This is not a one night or one week effect. It takes about 3 months for this effect on the blood pressure to manifest, so do not give up after one or two weeks and say there is no effect.

ACTION TIP

WALK 4 MILES EVERY DAY

15 Simple Ways To Lower Your Blood Pressure Naturally After 40 Without Complicated Diets

Reduce stress: Sleep well

Sleeping well will help you lower your blood pressure. As we get older we discover that sleep does not come as readily as in the past. Not sleeping well eventually affects your health. One way most people try to deal with insomnia is to take sleeping pills. However, another option is to increase the amount of physical exercise that you participate in during the day. This is one of the key ways to help you get a good sleep at night. The more active your body is during the day, the more likely you are to relax at night and fall asleep faster.

If you doubt this, watch your children. You will find out they sleep the most, when they have been most busy running around and actively playing all day. They get into bed and fall sound asleep.

15 Simple Ways To Lower Your Blood Pressure Naturally After 40 Without Complicated Diets

With regular exercise you'll notice that your quality of sleep is improved and the transition between the cycles and phases of sleep will become smoother and more regular. By keeping up your physical activity during the day, you may find it easier to deal with the stress and worries of your life.

Research and studies indicate that there is a direct correlation between how much we exercise and how we feel afterwards. You should try and increase your physical activity during the day. The goal here is to give your body enough stimulation during the day so that you aren't full of energy at night.

Your body requires a certain amount of physical activity in order to keep functioning in a healthy manner. It is also important to note that you should not be exercising one or two hours before you go to bed. Make your own individualized time-frame based on your experience.

The ideal exercise time is in the late afternoon or early evening. You want to make sure you expend your physical energy long before it is time for your body to rest and ready itself for sleep.

If you discover that you don't have any time to exercise on a regular basis, you should try to sneak in moments of physical activity into your daily schedule. Whenever possible, you should take the stairs instead of the elevator, and form the habit of walking around whenever it is safe to do so.

Apart from exercise, the other factors that contribute to poor sleep include watching too much TV and using your mobile devices late at night. Don't stay up late to watch your favorite show. You may enjoy your show but you will end up not sleeping well at night. This will not be good for your blood pressure especially if you are over 40 years old. Remember to turn off your computer and your mobile devices like your cell phone and IPAD. Your overall goal here is to have a deep and restful sleep of about 6 to 8 hours everyday.

ACTION TIPS

EXERCISE WELL DURING THE DAY
TURN OFF YOUR DEVICES

Improve your emotional well-being

Our emotional well-being is very important for our blood pressure because feeling good about ourselves reduces our daily stress level and helps to make our interactions with others more enjoyable. The more stress we have the more stress hormones we release in our bodies that will make our blood pressure shoot up.

There are factors and activities throughout the day that can affect our emotional well-being. These include time management, stress, relationship conflicts, anxiety and anger. The truth is that we all have problems or things we do not do well. Taking part in such activities can either lead to emotional tension or can lead others to stress you out, by reminding you of your inadequacies. Our emotions play a big role on how we respond to our daily circumstances. The compass method for emotional management encourages us to discover ourselves so that we can manage our emotions in a way that fits our inner self.

One of the best ways we can protect our emotional well-being and, by extension reduce our high blood pressure, is to expect the unexpected. Each one of us must find ways to deal with those times when people return kindness with rudeness, fairness with unfairness. Whenever I encounter such situations, I remind myself that how I react is more important than whatever is said by someone else.

One of the keys to improving emotional well-being and reducing blood pressure would be finding healthy ways to deal with our perception of our environment. This would include how we deal with our social and physical environment. This includes how we interact with others and how we deal with our deepest fears. If we don't get it right, we build up stress that will ultimately affect our sleep, heart and digestive systems. We all know that stress can cause high blood pressure, stomach ulcers and even sleepless nights.

We can empower ourselves to deal with such circumstances by changing our internal dialogue. As an example instead of saying, "I am not going to stay here and be insulted", you could remind yourself that people lash out or say mean things when they feel frustrated, insecure, uncomfortable or unappreciated. This is just an emotional outburst. Do not take such outbursts personal. Remember that nothing that exists is perfect.

Instead treat each outburst or episode as an opportunity to be thankful. One of the ways to empower yourself is to learn your emotional triggers and have strategies to deal with such situations before they arise or as soon as they arise. Self-knowledge, which is one of the seven dimensions of the compass health profile, will definitely enable us to empower ourselves and live more healthy lives.

ACTION TIP

IGNORE EMOTIONAL OUTBURSTS

Improve your emotional well-being: Manage your daily conflicts

One of the advantages of having an integrated mind set is that it allows you to look at conflicts as an opportunity for change and growth. Conflict resolution is a useful tool for reducing your blood pressure because it will help you reduce stress. It is a skill you can start to use for your daily life immediately.

Conflicts can teach us a lot about ourselves and how to become more competent and effective in our communications with others. This tool can also help us avoid relationship minefields because it helps each person to recognize behavior patterns that lead to conflict. It can help us reduce or even cut down on stress.

15 Simple Ways To Lower Your Blood Pressure Naturally After 40 Without Complicated Diets

Long standing conflicts indicate a growing need to change and an increasing resistance to doing so. They expose contradictory social messages, the absence of obvious vision, or the presence of blind spots. They indicate the moment of discovery that one finds out that something isn't working and the need for a fresh approach to fix or transcend it. The determining element in virtually every conflict resolution may be the mindset of the people involved and their desire to end the conflict. .

In a way this a very sophisticated way of saying that conflicts help us to realize the areas in our lives in which we need to change as well as those situations and circumstances that lead to a build up of stress in our relationships. Remember that the more you reduce stress the more your reduce blood pressure.

To some extent, our conflicts are due to our differing needs and wants. The husband might want to spend money and the wife might want to save it. At other times, it is between parents and their children. The child's need is to explore, so the street or the cliff fulfills a need. But the parents' need is to protect the child's safety, so limiting exploration turns into a bone of contention between them. Parents can make this a teachable moment by acknowledging the child's need to explore while encouraging the child to do it in a safer environment.

We all need to feel understood, nurtured, and helped, but the ways in which these wants are met vary broadly because of our different personalities and spiritual outlooks. Recognizing that conflicts are part of every relationship will help us not to take them too personal and use them as opportunities for growth and reduce emotional tension.

15 Simple Ways To Lower Your Blood Pressure Naturally After 40 Without Complicated Diets

How we feel affects how we see ourselves and how we interact with others. If we do not feel good about ourselves, we are less likely to do those things that will make us happy and healthy.

For example, being in a bad mood can make us decide to skip the fruits and salads that we know are good for our health. Worse still, you may feel so bad that you end up drinking and smoking.

If you feel sad and you skip your fruits and vegetables, you may end up eating your comfort food. This will make you gain weight or at least fail to lose weight. The more weight you gain the more work you give to your heart. This means giving your heart a bigger area to pump blood to. This will mean increasing your blood pressure. Sadly adding to your blood pressure as a hypertensive will only make matters worse.

15 Simple Ways To Lower Your Blood Pressure Naturally After 40 Without Complicated Diets

If you are dealing with negative feelings, counter them by going through thoughts of thankfulness. This approach will help you to find much more positive thoughts. Positive thoughts will lead to positive feelings and positive action.

For each negative feeling, find and say 10 thankful thoughts or things you are most thankful for. You could be thankful because you are alive, or thankful for your children or even thankful that you are looking for ways to reduce your blood pressure and depend less on medications.

ACTION TIP

FIND AND SAY 10 THANKFUL THOUGHTS EVERYDAY

15 Simple Ways To Lower Your Blood Pressure Naturally After 40 Without Complicated Diets

Improve your daily emotional well-being: Maintain balance

If you are hypertensive, you have very little margin for error. Daily emotional tension which is usually as a result of emotional imbalance can increase your blood pressure and lead to more damage to your body. This is why maintaining your emotional well-being through balanced living is a very important of reducing your blood pressure naturally.

Balance is an important part of the Compass method for lowering your blood pressure. Maintaining the balance that we need to live healthy is not easy for most of us. Although balance is desired, it is hard to achieve because we are discouraged by the pain necessary for change and growth. One of the reasons this happens is that

15 Simple Ways To Lower Your Blood Pressure Naturally After 40 Without Complicated Diets

we look at the magnitude of the change desired instead of the small steps we can take to achieve the balance we need for growth in our lives.

Stress builds up because our expectations become more than the results that we can get. We expect 100% good relationships all the time, yet in the end we would be lucky to get 50% good relationships. We forget that nobody is perfect and fail to maintain the balance between our work and relationships. We sometimes put in 80% of our energy into work, and 20% of our energy into our relationships and we still expect our relationships to be stellar. When our relationships struggle we become frustrated and stressed out.

We allow ourselves to be defined by our work. Jesus was a carpenter but Jesus was defined by his spirituality and relationship with others through which He radiated balance and mastery of life. If you are a person of faith you can learn from this.

15 Simple Ways To Lower Your Blood Pressure Naturally After 40 Without Complicated Diets

If we fail to strike the right balance between our work and our relationships then there will be a build up of stress and illness in our lives. We shall find ourselves quick to anger and less tolerant of others and their mistakes. We shall find ourselves less able to concentrate and enjoy the simple pleasures of daily life.

Part of the reason this happens is because you have failed to deliver on expectations. Remember when expectations fail to match results, stress arises. Self-reflection and meditation will help us to identify the areas of our lives that are growing too fast as we seek to find balance in our lives. It will also help us learn to forgive ourselves and others. We can make modifications that will enable us to grow without crashing. Having uncontrolled high blood pressure, with stroke or heart attack can lead to a bad crash.

15 Simple Ways To Lower Your Blood Pressure Naturally After 40 Without Complicated Diets

How much balance do you have in your life? Is your triangle of happiness balanced? To find out how much balance you have in your life spend fifteen minutes of your day, examining how much time you spend on your finances, relationships, and health . This type of examination is an important aspect of self-knowledge which is important for your growth and spiritual health.

This is only the first step in our trying to find balance in our lives. It is an important first step because it allows us to examine our relations, health habits, and finances and determine which aspects require more time and more improvement.

ACTION TIPS

LOWER YOUR EXPECTATIONS FROM OTHERS

FORGIVE AND FORGIVE AGAIN

Improve your daily emotional well- being: Change the negative patterns that dominate your life

Another way to improve your daily emotional well-being is to change the negative patterns that occur most frequently in your daily life. It is now an accepted notion that a person's social life can have a big impact on the state of his or her health or happiness. People who spend a lot of time being social have a healthier and longer life than those who keep themselves isolated. This is another of those changes that is always possible to make. Try to find activities that you enjoy and that allow you to socialize.

Examine the past 48 hours of your life and see the situations and circumstances that predominantly make you unhappy. These are negative patterns that lead to stress, emotional tension, poor emotional control and unhappiness.

A common pattern, I had to overcome was "list overloading". I had the tendency to list too many things I wanted to do everyday. Sometimes I had a long list like 10 things, without taking into account how long each item would take.

The end result would be that halfway through the day, I would realize that I could not get all I wanted to do, done. This had the effect of making me feel bad about myself. I would begin to feel that I had not worked hard enough to accomplish the simple tasks I had set out for myself just for one day.

I would get stressed out and feel that the only way out would be to take a time out and eat some food. Yes, eat some food to relax! In such negative moments, I would just grab a soda and some snacks which I would just gobble down my throat to help me feel better.

Well, you can imagine how that has helped my "healthy" eating plan. This simply made me gain more weight and give my heart more work to do. Giving your heart more work to do is the last thing you want to do as a hypertensive.

It took me a while to realize that the problem was not the soda and snacks, but it had more to do with my emotional stress resulting from my poor planning for the day. If you are over 40 and hypertensive, there are a number of daily activities or challenges that are stress generators or "list busters" Here are a few examples of stress generators:

15 Simple Ways To Lower Your Blood Pressure Naturally After 40 Without Complicated Diets

Your teenage daughter won't listen to you anymore

You were passed over for a promotion

You mother in-law came to visit

You had your second accident for the year

You still haven't been able to quit smoking

Your husband never listens to you

Your wife complains about everything you do

Your husband went out drinking with boys again

You still haven't fixed the lawn mower

Your car won't start this morning

You forget your anniversary

These days, I make my list for the day and attach a time frame to it so that I have an idea about how much time I shall put into each block of activity. I also divide my list into non-urgent, urgent and immediate projects. Immediate projects get done first and others follow.

This approach has helped me cut down on the emotional stress that my past pattern of negativity generated. It is a welcome experience because it has helped cut down on my episodes of emotional eating.

According to a study from the University of Alabama, those who ate in response to an emotional stress-were 13 times more likely to be overweight or obese. We all know the additional health risks associated with being overweight.

The advantage of recognizing the patterns that dominate your life negatively is that you can either change them or be better prepared to respond to such stressors when they occur .While you are in the process of changing these negative patterns that dominate your life, create an automatic response that you can use in such situations without having to eat food.

An example would be to chew bubble gum, when you feel emotionally stressed instead of drinking soda and taking snacks. If you do not like bubble gums, drink water or eat an apple. Of course it depends on what you are dealing with. I am not sure chewing bubble gum will help deal with stress from your mother in law's visit. One way to deal with type of stress is to find excuses to leave the house frequently. Live to fight another day! Sometimes in order to protect your health, you have to take a short gap measure until you can develop a long-term strategy to deal with recurring negative patterns.

ACTION TIPS

MAKE A LIST WITH A TIME FRAME RECOGNIZE YOUR NEGATIVE PATTERN STRESS GENERATORS

Lose weight: Reduce your waist line

If you reduce your waistline, you will reduce your blood pressure. This is because an increase in waist line is usually associated with an increase in your body surface area and weight. This means you heart has a larger area to distribute blood to, and requires a higher blood pressure to do so.

As you get older you begin to notice a tiny but perceptible bulge in your waist line. At first you try to ignore it because you know, you haven't changed your eating habits or daily routine. Yet the bulge continues to grow. Sadly at 40, most people are old enough to notice this type of bulge and increase in waist line.

While a few people look at the bulge as a sign good living majority consider it as an embarrassing sign of aging. Knowing why you have the bulge will help you to be more motivated to reduce it. Remember that for men the waist circumference measured above the hip bones while relaxed and exhaling should not be more than 40 inches or 100cm and for women not more than 35 inches or 88cm.The exception is pregnancy for woman.

One of the main reasons why our belly fat increases after 40 is because our muscle mass decreases with age. When this happens our ability to use up energy becomes decreased so that the unused energy becomes converted into visceral fat in our internal organs leading to the belly bulge.

The second reason is that we get older we have more new sources of stress. You now have to worry about your job, your mortgage, your children's education and your in-laws. New sources of stress mean more release of cortisol, the stress hormone. Cortisol leads to the distribution of fat into the abdominal area, making a bad situation worse. Cortisol will also cause the retention of sodium and will lead to increased blood volume. Increase in blood volume will lead to a proportionate increase in blood pressure.

Knowing at least these two reasons, you will now look at your belly fat more like a health-marker than as a cosmetic problem and will want to reduce your belly fat fast. Sadly you will discover that the bulge or belly fat is not easy to get rid of. If you have tried to get rid of your own bulge, I am sure you would agree with me.

I will share with you how I lost weight in six weeks, I lost 10 pounds in six weeks by eating plenty of vegetables and fruits while reducing my food portion per meal by about a half and walking for at least 45 minutes, at least five times a week. I started by walking 30 minutes a day for the first week, then I increased it to 45 minutes a day.

15 Simple Ways To Lower Your Blood Pressure Naturally After 40 Without Complicated Diets

After about 6 weeks, I found it difficult to consistently create the 45 minutes block of time, so I changed to 3 blocks of 15 minute-time intervals everyday. The advantage of this approach, which is one of the cornerstones of the compass method, was that it was gradual and I slowly incorporated it into my lifestyle. It has also helped me to reduce my waist line and gain better control of my blood pressure.

To trim your waistline faster, you need to include exercises that will further strengthen your muscles. This is important because after 40 years of age, muscle strength becomes weaker. If you fail to take action to strengthen your muscles, you will end up with a more protruding belly. You can do this by participating in muscle strengthening activities like playing tennis, doing pushups and jump ropes every week. Choose one of these or any other similar one that will work best for your personality, experience and schedule and do it regularly.

I will share with you Ray's method for doing muscle strengthening. Ray is a friend of mine who uses his own unique combination of pushups to tone his muscles. It consists doing at least 50 pushups every day. However, he does it by doing 10 pushups at a time. After each ten, take a 1 to 3 minute break, then continue until you have completed 50 pushups. If you cannot do it all in one session break it up into two or three sessions that you find comfortable. If 50 a day is too high a target for you, start with 20 a day. Do not exceed 50 a day and do you pushups on alternate days, to give your muscles time to recover and grow.

These muscle-strengthening exercises will help your increase your muscle mass as well as increase your total energy expenditure and reduce the amount of excess energy to be converted to visceral or stomach fat. No matter which muscle strengthening exercise you decide to use, take time to draw your own weight loss pie chart. It will help you monitor your progress.

Weight Loss In A Pie Chart

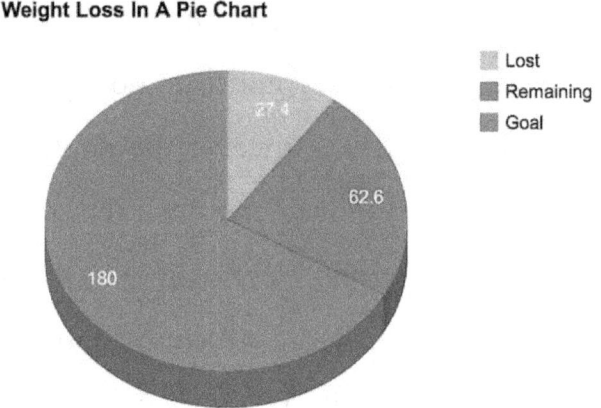

This picture is from Laurence Simon from Flickr.com

ACTION TIP

MEASURE YOUR WAIST CIRCUMFERENCE

Lose weight: Make losing weight fun

If you want to lose weight in a manner that will last, you have to make losing weight fun. If not you will start then stop. Sometimes, I have to chuckle at how we concentrate too much on the total amount of pounds we have to lose, instead of finding simple and easy ways to lose a few pounds per week.

Once you discover what works for you that you can do consistently, your weight loss will occur naturally. This way you will find yourself also reducing your blood pressure gradually. **By following the approaches discussed so far in this book you will discover your own individualized plan that is fun for you**.

First, be realistic do not try to lose 100 pounds in two days or one week. This is very hard to do in an enjoyable and practical manner. Losing weight is not the same as starvation. A more realistic goal might be losing 10 pounds in one month or 6 weeks.

Second, remember the reason why you want to lose weight. It is because you want to lower your blood pressure so that you can reduce your chances of having complications that can seriously damage your health and reduce your quality of life. You already know that you do not want to spend your old age in nursing homes suffering from one chronic illness after another. You want to have fun and age gracefully.

Third, do not worry about results. Concentrate on actually doing or taking the steps you set up in your simple plan for losing weight. If your plan requires walking 45 minutes a day, do it. Do not make excuses. If you are too busy to spare chunks of 45 minutes at a time, then cut it down to 15 minutes at a time.

Fourth, do not think like a child. Do not think that it is either you are getting everything right or everything is wrong. If you plan to walk 45 minutes a day but due to circumstances beyond your control you were able to do only 20 minutes, you have not failed. Do the 20 minutes that day, then do 70 minutes the next day. This still makes a total of 90 minutes in two days. On the third day you can go back to 45 minutes a day. Be flexible.

Fifth, make sure you keep track of your progress. Weigh yourself before you start then weigh yourself after every week. You can use a simple scale to weigh yourself. If you want something a little more comprehensive, you can calculate your BMI (Body Mass Index), by measuring your height as well. The next step would be to put your height, weight, age and sex, into a BMI calculator and you would find out your BMI. Normal BMI is between 18.5 and 24.9. The advantage of taking measurements is that it gives you an easy way of checking how much progress you have made. When you check that scale and discover that you have actually met your first realistic goal, the smile on your face will encourage you to keep on trying. You will become more energized.

These are five fun ways to lose weight. Losing weight and maintaining your weight within the normal range for your age and height is certainly one of the ways to lower your blood pressure.

ACTION TIP

FIND OUT OR CALCULATE YOUR BMI

Lose weight: Measure your weight every week

Measuring your weight regularly is one of the easiest check on how your individualized health plan is working. It is easier to do than calculating your BMI or measuring your waist circumference. Just climb on a scale and read your weight. The last time I checked my weight, I discovered that I had gained back some weight.

This made me do a mental review of the week I discovered that I had a problem with snacks. I eat too much snack at night when I did feel like sleeping though I needed to be sleeping. My solution was eat more snacks late at night.. This is an ongoing challenge. This Was I bad idea and I find out early because I had formed the habit of weighing myself every week. This I was able to catch my weight gain and go back to my own individualized plan for weight loss. I replaced the late night snacks with nuts and banana.

As a hypertensive, you have to remember that you have less room for error, because high blood pressure already puts a lot of tension on your heart, vessels and vital organs. If you fail to deal with daily stress well, you will get sad and depressed and you will end up attempting to eat or snack to deal with it. This will slowly lead you to gaining back weight you had previously lost. This will occur gradually and you can only catch it early if you weigh yourself every week. This you can take small steps quickly lose the weight you have gained. If you do not weigh yourself weekly by the time you discover your new weight gain, it will be too late to lose it fast. Meanwhile you putting more pressure on your heart and increasing your chances of having complications.

15 Simple Ways To Lower Your Blood Pressure Naturally After 40 Without Complicated Diets

Here are a few tips to help you lose weight and prevent these potential life-altering complications. First, remember to do your 72- hour life activity review to find out if there is anything bothering you in your relationships, health, or work. If you are diabetic and you do not know it, you cannot effectively address your weight problem until you see a specialist for your diabetes.

All things being equal, if you discover that you have been gaining weight back simply because you couldn't stick to your individual health plan, then here are a few more tips for you to consider.

A lapse is not a relapse. A mistake is not a failure. If you find yourself not sticking to your fruits and vegetables, think about trying out new fruits that you have not tried in the past. Talk to your support group, and share your ideas on eating time and food variety. Try again if you do not succeed the first time. If you are living by yourself and are longer in touch with your family or old friends, create a new support group or join on online. Become more active in your community. Volunteer in the church or other societies that you belong to.

Finally, do not forget to talk to your doctor or health care provider about your medications. Make sure you are not taking any medications that may make you gain weight. This is particularly important if through a chart of your weekly weight measurement you discover you have either been gaining weight or not losing as much as you expected.

ACTION TIPS

A LAPSE IS A NOT A RELAPSE

WEIGH YOURSELF EVERY WEEK

Miscellaneous: Laugh more often

The more you laugh, the more you relax. The more you relax, the more you reduce tension and stress. This will help to reduce your blood pressure. You have to learn to use laughter to deal with stress in your everyday life. You can decide the best time for you to do your laughing. You can consider it your "laughter therapy time".

A common question I get, when I tell people about "laughter therapy time" is "How do I make myself laugh during that period?" Think of all the activities that made you laugh in the past and in the past 72 hours. They could be your past mistakes or funny family accidents.

15 Simple Ways To Lower Your Blood Pressure Naturally After 40 Without Complicated Diets

The benefits of laughing are many. It helps you feel good about yourself. It uplifts your mood and helps to lower your stress level and blood pressure.

Creating five-minute periods of "laughter therapy time" loosens tension and uplifts our moods. You can do this at end of the day or during the middle of a heated argument with your spouse, friend or colleague. This will give you a chance to step back and remind yourself that "It could have been worse."

I share this idea with you because I have found it very useful in the past. It has stopped me from going off on a tirade on a number of times and saved my heart and lungs from the consequences of the stress-related hormonal surges.

Laughter is indeed the best medicine. Laugh a little, laugh often, it will make you feel good about yourself and reduce the chances that you will engage in negative health activity like binge drinking or eating. Emotional eating can lead to over snacking and can hinder you from keeping off weight even after having a good start.

Try to spend more time with people that make you laugh. Do not let isolated live events make you isolate yourself and spend less time with people that love your company. Sadly after Tom lost his job he found himself spending less time with his kids. Inadvertently, he also cut down on his laughter time. I told him to go back to having a laughter period with his kids. I encouraged him to find out from his kids the fun and funny activities and events that happened to them everyday.

Initially, Tom said he could not to do it every day because he was mad at the world following his job loss. The problem was that he had noticed that his blood pressure had started to go up. I encouraged him to set aside one day of the week for everyone in the family to share with others the seven funniest things that had happened to them over the week. After initially refusing he reluctantly agreed to do it.

Four weeks later, Tom told me he had rediscovered his joy. He said he started feeling better after he started spending about 1 hour every Sunday laughing with his family. They laughed over their list of their seven funniest activities for the week. He was surprised to find out that having this laughter period helped him to feel good about himself, though he still had no job. This helped him to reverse the upward trend in his blood pressure.

In addition to getting his blood pressure lower, Tom became more confident and he slowly stopped being mad at the world. He became more positive about the future. You too can use the funniest events of the week to create your own "laughter therapy time" and make your life healthier.

ACTION TIP

LAUGH MORE OFTEN EVERYDAY

15 Simple Ways To Lower Your Blood Pressure Naturally After 40 Without Complicated Diets

Miscellaneous: Quit smoking

Stopping smoking can help you reduce your risk of heart problems, stroke, high blood pressure, lung cancer, and even breathing complications. According to the Mayo Clinic, smoking increases your blood pressure and also damages your arteries. Remember that after quitting smoking you are able to reverse many of the harmful effects of cigarettes, no matter how long you have been a smoker.

For example, if you quit smoking for a period of 5 years, you are no more at risk of a stroke than someone who has been a non-smoker for their entire life. This is huge considering that those who smoke are considered at least twice as likely to suffer a stroke. Additionally, if you quit for 15 years, you can enjoy the same risk of coronary heart disease as a non-smoker. While it might seem strange to enjoy the risk for coronary heart disease, it is much better than actually having coronary heart disease. Taking these small victories for your health is important since you will be able to significantly improve your quality of life.

Not everyone is concerned about the health benefits. If you find yourself more concerned with the money, then focus on what you can save. Ultimately, the reason you choose to quit smoking is up to you. The way you do it will be based on your personality and smoking habits. You need to look at your lifestyle and determine what truly matters for you. If you are more determined to improve your health then focus your efforts on the health benefits that stopping smoking for good can really have for you.

Alternatively you may want to quit because smoking is causing problems like asthma for your children. You may want to quit so that you can do better when run with your kids, play with friends or just simply to get rid of the smell and unkempt appearance associated with smoking.

Remember when it was culturally acceptable to smoke cigarettes everywhere. Now you cannot smoke cigarettes in bars, planes, airport terminals and office buildings. If you have forgotten, watch movies from the 1930's to the 1970's. What if you were one of the few to have questioned the cultural norm of smoking everywhere? You would have tried to protect your health even before the policies that banned smoking became the law.

Do not let your fear of what others will say to discourage you. The good thing is that no matter your reason for quitting smoking the positive impact on your blood pressure will remain.

ACTION TIPS

FOCUS ON ONE MOTIVATION AT A TIME

QUIT SMOKING

Miscellaneous: Recognize financial stress

Since financial issues and problems are an important part of life after age 40, it is important to recognize financial stress as a real threat to your blood pressure and your health. Remember that we need money to pay for mortgage, send our kids to college and hang out with friends. We also need money to buy healthy food, to go to the laboratory for tests or doctor's visits, go to the movies and even to sign up for gym membership.

Not having finances to pay your rent or your mortgage could result in losing your home. Just worrying about how to take care of these bills can be lead to stress. You have to remember that no matter the source of stress, whether it is physical, physiological or psychological, chronic stress will eventually lead to damage to your heart, vessels and other organs.

This is one of the reasons why it is important that when you are examining your ambition and self-knowledge profile, you should be try as much as possible to estimate how much you earn and how you will spend it. Remember that if you are retired, there is a fixed income, you get every month. Plan your budget accordingly and be selective on how you spend your money.

Worrying about money issues can build up your pressure? Worse still, the chronic state of sympathetic elevation caused by adrenaline can lead to arrhythmias (fast irregular heartbeats) and sudden death. Do not try to solve all your financial problems at once. Set up a plan to deal with your financial challenges one step at a time.

15 Simple Ways To Lower Your Blood Pressure Naturally After 40 Without Complicated Diets

The state of your finances or unstable financial situation could significantly affect your ability to implement your individualized compass health plan. If you are concerned about your finances, talk to a financial expert or talk to trusted friends and family members who have a track record of handling their finances well. Do not talk to someone you do not trust because some scam artists will only make matters worse.

At least having a financial plan will help to reduce the stress that comes from not knowing what to do. The case of my patient who suffered from sleepless nights made me to appreciate the link between finances and good health. Her problems started when those who were supposed to help her get a loan modification ruined her credit and almost cost her, her home.

15 Simple Ways To Lower Your Blood Pressure Naturally After 40 Without Complicated Diets

Her life changed from having sound sleep every night to sleepless nights. When I used my findings in her comprehensive health assessment protocol to check her triangle of happiness, I found out about her financial worries. I told her that the first step she needed to take was to spend what little money she had smartly and wisely. For example, I told her she could start saving money by buying things with coupons more regularly.

Of course, I also strongly encouraged her to see a financial expert to resolve her financial worries. I cannot give you details of what her own financial plan was, but I know that she resolved her financial stress and had more peaceful sleep. Don't ignore your finances and learn to live within your means while planning for the future.

This approach will help you to cut down on stress, sleep more soundly and reduce your blood pressure. You will more time to spend doing the things you love doing, instead of worrying about medications and their side effects. You will have more time to spend with your loved ones and friends, than with your doctors.

ACTION TIP

HAVE A THIRD-PATHWAY INDEPENDENT FINANCIAL PLAN

15 Simple Ways To Lower Your Blood Pressure Naturally After 40 Without Complicated Diets

Miscellaneous: Support yourself with supplements

Take your daily multivitamin supplements but do not let them replace your healthy habits. For example take your omega 3 and 6 fatty acids which have been proven to be very helpful for the heart and in lowering blood pressure. However do not give up on fish just because you take Omega fatty acids. You may need to talk to your doctor before you start taking Omega fatty acids especially if you are on Coumadin, aspirin or ginkgo. Why? This is because there may be an increased risk of bleeding with high doses of Omega 3 fatty acids which can be made worse by blood thinners like Coumadin.

Remember that lowering your blood pressure naturally depends on forming and maintaining

15 Simple Ways To Lower Your Blood Pressure Naturally After 40 Without Complicated Diets

good relationships and habits that will help you deal with daily stress and unexpected life events. Do not forget that "He who fails to prepare, prepares to fail".

Taking your multivitamins should not stop you from going for your regular medical checkup as recommended for your age group and family history by your doctor or health care provider.

Find out what you need to do and then do it. If you need to get vaccines, get your vaccines like the flu vaccines. Do not just say you are taking vitamin C and refuse to take vaccines and exercise. If you need to bundle up because it is cold, do it. Wash your hands frequently to minimize your chances of getting an infection.

It is a huge mistake to assume that simply because you use multivitamins you will remain perfectly healthy or suffer only mild illness. Remember that vitamins are usually supplemental and your taking daily multivitamins will be most effective only if you continue to eat healthy, exercise regularly and continue to manage your weight and the sources of daily stress in your life.

Eating right, means that in addition to taking multivitamins, you also make sure you eat fruits and vegetables. The good thing about this, is that through fruits and vegetables, you will also get phytochemicals and fiber in their most natural form.

The conventional recommendation in this regard is to eat at least five servings of vegetables and fruits per day. One way to do this, is to eat plenty of fruits and vegetables servings, per meal every day then use fruits like Persian cucumber or apples for snacks. You can eat Persian cucumbers directly, or simply cut them up and put them in main dishes as a salad. This can easily get you to the five servings per day goal. Another way, you can increase your fruits and vegetables intake would be by making half of the plate in each meal filled with fruits and vegetables or taking an apple per meal.

Eat your fruits and vegetables every day, but make sure you start your day with your daily dose of your preferred multivitamins without allowing them to supplant the healthy habits you have acquired or are in the process of acquiring.

For example, we know that vitamin B can be found in fish, meat, orange juice and fortified cereals, yet we also know we do not always get to eat enough of the food types I have just listed. If you combine trying to eat right with taking your vitamins, you would end up regularly getting enough vitamin B in your body. This is an example of how you can use vitamins as a health supplement.

Why are B vitamins so important? Because they help to lower the level of homocysteine in blood vessels, which at high levels can lead to damage of the lining of arteries and could lead to a faster formation of blood clots.

Other vitamins that have been specifically linked to the heart and to lowering blood pressure are vitamin D, Omega-3 fatty acids and Coenzyme 10 or CQ10. CQ10 is an antioxidant that is highly concentrated in heart muscle.

CQ10 cardiac effects include helping to lower blood pressure. According to Prof. Frank Rosenfeldt of Monash University in Australia, CQ10 has the potential in patients with high blood pressure to lower diastolic blood pressure by up to

10mm Hg and systolic pressure by 17mm Hg with little side effects. According to Bradley Tompkins in the *Life extension magazine*, the other cardiac benefit is that CQ10 helps to improve the survival of patients with severe heart failure.

CQ10 levels are reduced by statins and aging. If you are on statins ask your doctor about your CQ10 level. Those 20 years of age and above have reduced levels of CQ10. This does not mean that people over 40 should automatically take CQ10 supplements. It just means that your age and health condition are factors to consider when deciding whether to take or not to take CQ10.

ACTION TIP

TAKE APPROPRIATE SUPPLEMENTS DAILY

Miscellaneous: Become part of a group

Community relationships are important components of the Compass Method. Examine your relationship with yourself and with others. Do not try to do everything by yourself. Join a group or form one. This is because no man is an island. It does not have to be a formal group. It could easily be a group made up of family members or friends. Believe me, it is a lot of fun when the whole family is involved in healthy eating and healthy living activities like running and sports.

Making everybody in your family a part of your healthy living plan is a great idea. If you tell your children that you are no longer going to add salt to your meals, they will remind you if you forget and try to do it. They will keep you accountable.

15 Simple Ways To Lower Your Blood Pressure Naturally After 40 Without Complicated Diets

Another benefit, you get out of this, is that you start getting into the act of eating healthy. It will be easier to buy milk with reduced fat and get the whole family to eat small carrots and pomegranates.

The next people you need to get into your group will be those in your office whom you share a lunch break with. This way when you think of going for soda, candies and cookies, you will have someone reminding you that you have decided to eat fruits and vegetables during your lunch break. A salad is also a good way to go.

Depending on your budget and personality, you may want to try more formal groups than the ones I have mentioned above. These may be online or offline groups. Whatever group you decide to join, make sure you join a group that suits your personality, your budget and your time. Do not make becoming part of a group a new source of stress for you.

ACTION TIP

BECOME PART OF A GROUP OR A TEAM

15 Simple Ways To Lower Your Blood Pressure Naturally After 40 Without Complicated Diets

Don't forget your spirituality

You can use spirituality to reduce your blood pressure. Talking about spirituality is usually challenging because it be divisive. Electronic gadgets and easily available multiple entertainment sources also lead most of to focus mostly on our physical wants and needs. If you can strike the balance between the material and spiritual aspects of your life you will have even more ways to deal with stress and improve yourself.

Looking at the spiritual aspect of your life will mean that you will be prepared to look closely and reflect on your thoughts, feelings, beliefs, and motivations. Intermittently examining your experiences, the decisions you make, the relationships you have, and the things you have will help you do this. Remember to forgive yourself and others.

15 Simple Ways To Lower Your Blood Pressure Naturally After 40 Without Complicated Diets

There are differences in opinion about what spirituality means. Religion and science have differing views on matters of the human spirit. Religion views people as spiritual beings temporarily living on Earth, while science views the spirit as just one dimension of an individual. Mastery of the self is a recurring theme in both Western and Eastern teachings. The needs of the body are recognized but placed under the needs of the spirit. Beliefs, values, morality, rules, experiences, and good works provide the blueprint to ensure the growth of the spiritual being.

In Psychology, realizing one's full potential is to self-actualize. Maslow identified several human needs: physiological, security, belongingness, esteem, cognitive, aesthetic, self-actualization, and self-transcendence. These needs can be categorized into material, emotional, and spiritual. When you have satisfied the basic physiological and emotional needs, spiritual or existential needs come next. Achieving each need leads to the total development of the individual.

The more you achieve the development of yourself the more you can gain a better understanding of the purpose of your life. As we discover this meaning, there are certain beliefs and values that we reject and affirm. Our lives have purpose. This purpose puts all our physical, emotional, and intellectual potentials into use; sustains us during trying times; and gives us something to look forward to---a goal to achieve, a destination to reach. A person without purpose or meaning is like a drifting boat in the ocean.

Knowing your purpose will help you to focus on the task at hand. It will also help us appreciate more the connections between everything. In psychology, connectedness is a characteristic of self-transcendence, the highest human need according to Maslow. Recognizing your connection to all things makes you more humble and respectful of people, animals, plants, and things in nature. It makes you appreciate everything around you. It moves you to go beyond your comfort zone and reach out to other people, and become stewards of all other things around you. This will also make you manage your blood pressure better because you will deal better with the unexpected experiences of daily life.

You have to realize that spiritual growth is a process that occurs day by day. We win some, we lose some, but the important thing is that we learn from our mistakes and continue to try to improve. Do not lose sight of this as you continue to strive to reduce your blood pressure naturally.

ACTION TIP

USE SPIRITUALITY YOUR OWN WAY

Conclusion

Don't give up even if you face challenges at the beginning. Cut down on sugars and processed foods. **Have an alternative food snack largely made of nuts and berries for when food cravings come while you are adjusting your diet**. Change takes time, be patient. **Growth is a process.**

Eat more berries, celery, garlic, bananas, pomegranates, fish, beans, dark chocolate and brown rice. **Reduce your food portion, increase your vegetables and fruits.** Eat an apple per meal and drink 2 glasses of water per meal.

Exercise everyday. **Walk 4 miles everyday** and do your pushups and jump ropes. Communicate better.

Reduce stress by talking strategically with others. Take a deep breath and sleep well everyday. Play, pray and meditate. Don't be afraid to be great. **Ask yourself what is controlling your thoughts?**

Daily action tips

UNDERSTAND YOURSELF BETTER

KNOW YOUR PASSION

ADJUST YOUR DAILY FOOD

DO A 72-HOUR FOOD AUDIT

CUT DOWN YOUR SERVING PORTIONS

EAT FOOD RICH IN FRUITS AND WHOLE GRAINS

MODIFY YOUR TYPICAL CULTURAL FOOD

DRINK TWO GLASSES OF WATER BEFORE EVERY MEAL

BALANCE YOUR DAILY FOOD TYPES

PLAN FOR YOUR SNACKS

CUTDOWN ON SODA AND BEER

READ YOUR NUTRITION FACTS

REDUCE SODIUM INTAKE

FOCUS ON EATING AND EAT SLOWLY

COOK WITH OLIVE OIL

EAT POMEGRANATES

EAT YOGURTS AND DARK CHOCOLATE

EAT CELERY

EAT BANANA AND CELERY

EAT TOMATOES

MANAGE YOUR CONVERSATIONS:

FOCUS ON THE BIG ROCKS

YOU DON'T HAVE TO HAVE THE LAST WORD

EXERCISE EVERYDAY:

15 Simple Ways To Lower Your Blood Pressure Naturally After 40 Without Complicated Diets

WALK 4 MILES EVERY DAY

SLEEP WELL

TURN OFF YOUR DEVICES

IMPROVE YOUR EMOTIONAL WELL-BEING

IGNORE EMOTIONAL OUTBURSTS

LOWER YOUR EXPECTATIONS FROM OTHERS

FORGIVE AND FORGIVE AGAIN

FIND AND SAY 10 THANKFUL THOUGHTS EVERYDAY

RECOGNIZE YOUR NEGATIVE PATTERN STRESS GENERATORS

MEASURE YOUR WAIST CIRCUMFERENCE

FIND OUT OR CALCULATE YOUR BMI

A LAPSE IS A NOT A RELAPSE

WEIGH YOURSELF EVERY WEEK

QUIT SMOKING

HAVE A THIRD-PATHWAY INDEPENDENT FINANCIAL PLAN

TAKE APPROPRIATE SUPPLEMENTS DAILY

BECOME PART OF A GROUP OR A TEAM

USE SPIRITUALITY YOUR OWN WAY

Appendix

DEVELOP YOUR OWN INDIVIDUALIZED BLUE PRINT FOR REDUCING BLOOD PRESSURE NATURALLY BASED ON THE COMPASS METHOD

If you have any questions contact me through www.compasswellnessinstitute.com

What will you do if your diet adjustment strategy fails or you cannot sustain your daily exercise regimen?

Do not give up. Reduce it to what you can do. If you cannot walk 4 miles a day, start with 1 mile a day. Build up slowly.

If you cannot cut down your food portion by half, cut it down by a quarter or by a third.

Add fruits and nuts slowly while you reduce your sodium and sugar intake.

Remember that sustainable change is a slow process. Do not give up on yourself. Don't

forget to always consult your doctor and keep your appointments.

Notes

American Journal of Clinical Nutrition

American Heart Association

Boyle, Marie, A. &Long, Sarah. 2010 *Personal*

   Nutrition. Wadsworth, Cengage learning

Bradley Tompkins, 2014, Life Extension

   Magazine. Retrieved from
   http://www.lifeextension.com/magazine/2
   014/4/coq10-proven-benefits-in-heart-
   failure-patients/page-01

CDC2015 High blood pressure retrieved from

   http://www.cdc.gov/bloodpressure/

Mayo Clinic 2015 High blood pressure (

   Hypertension):Causes Retrieved from
   http://www.mayoclinic.org/diseases-
   conditions/high-blood-
   pressure/basics/causes/con-20019580

National Institutes of Health (NIH)(2013)

Malignant Hypertension. *Medline Plus* Retrieved from http://www.nlm.nih.gov/medlineplus/ency/article/000491.htm

Nutrition Research

PLOS ONE

World Health Organization (WHO)(2015)

Global Health Observatory(GHO)data:

Blood Pressure. Retrieved from

http://www.who.int/gho/ncd/risk_factors/blood_pressure_prevalence/en/

Resources

Here are additional resources that will help you live a healthy, happy and successful life.

www.compasswellnessinstitute.com

www.compasshealthtransformer.com/members

www.dcompassmarketing.com

www.amenfathermbaka.com

http://www.amazon.com/Dr.-Chio-Ugochukwu/e/B00JNFLPQQ

Other books by Dr. Chio Ugochukwu include;

Too Young To Die

Praying To Win

The Compass Health Transformer: Your 72 Hour Blue Print For Healthy Living

21 Ways To Transform Your Health Without Medications

15 Simple Ways To Lower Your Blood Pressure Naturally After 40 Without Complicated Diets

The Compass Health Transformer Quit Smoking

The Compass Method for Weight Loss

Overcoming Daily Stress: 21 Quick And Easy Ways To Stay Stress-Free In Your Daily Life

The Secret To Daily happiness

Managing Time For Success

To order new or additional copies, please visit:

http://www.amazon.com/Dr.-Chio-Ugochukwu/e/B00JNFLPQQ

Call:661 992 6436

You can also get EBOOKS from

www.compasswellnessinstitute.com/Ebooks

About the Author

Dr. Chio Ugochukwu has always been interested in helping people improve their health, transform and become the best versions of themselves. He created the Transformational Abundant Living System (TALS) and developed the Compass Method to help individuals stay healthy and become more. He founded the Compass Research Institute to help individuals and organizations, maximize their strengths and overcome their weaknesses to get the best performance out of themselves, and become more empowered in their search for better health, more success and greater happiness despite their busy schedules, daily activities and duties.

He was inspired to create the TALS and the Compass Method, through the challenges he has encountered in his journey of life, his practice of medicine and his fascination with how the mind, the spirit and human experience influence the fulfillment of life. TALS is available at www.compasswellnessinstitute.com.

As an author and researcher, he has published many books, with peer-reviewed publications on quality of life and numerous articles on transformational living. He is the medical director of Dala Compass Foundation and a consultant with the Compass Research Institute. As a life-long learner, He is focused on sharing with individuals and organizations, customized methods and strategic pathways for getting the best performance for themselves and their organizations.

www.ingramcontent.com/pod-product-compliance
Lightning Source LLC
Chambersburg PA
CBHW070911290526
45795CB00001B/281